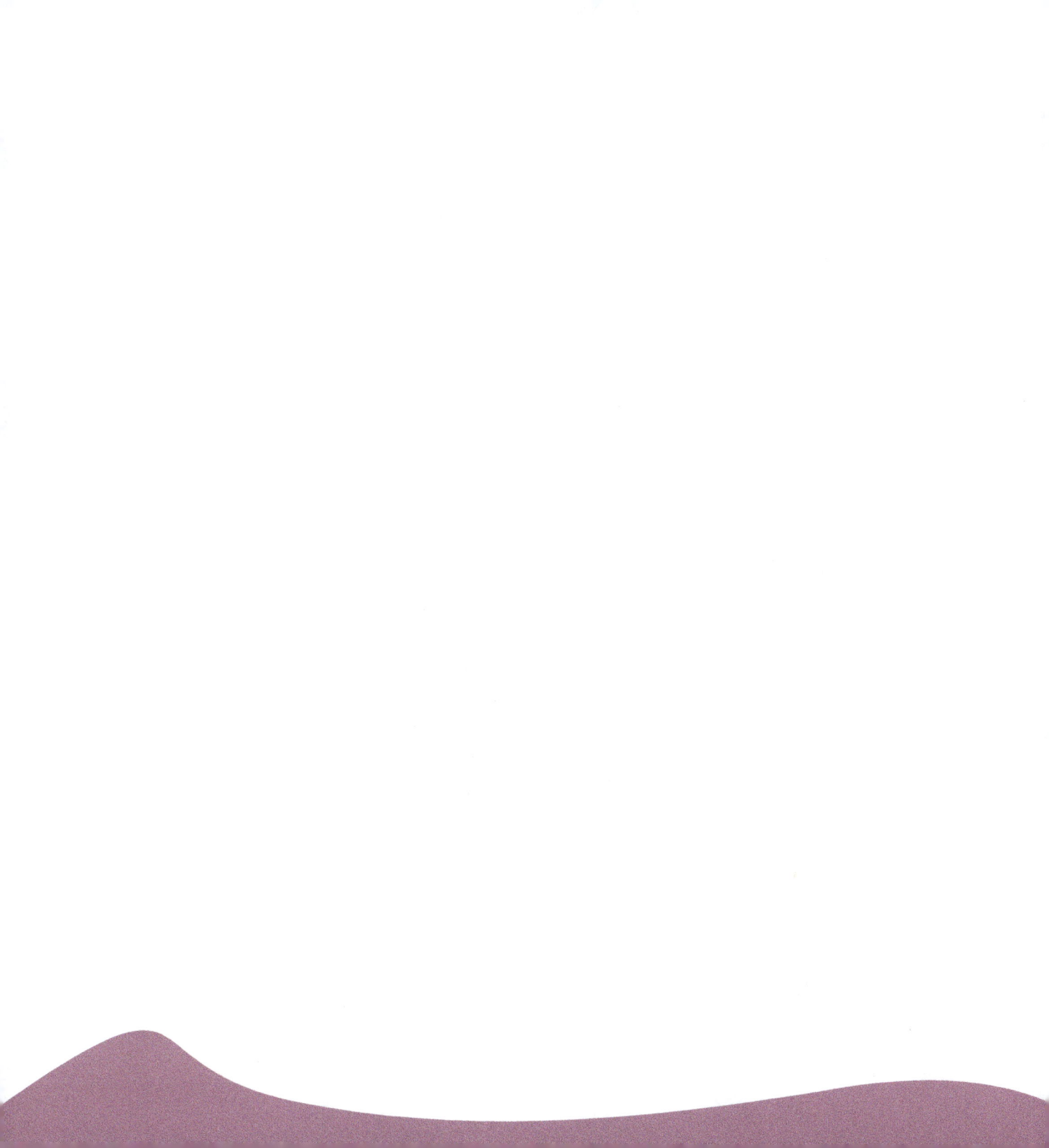

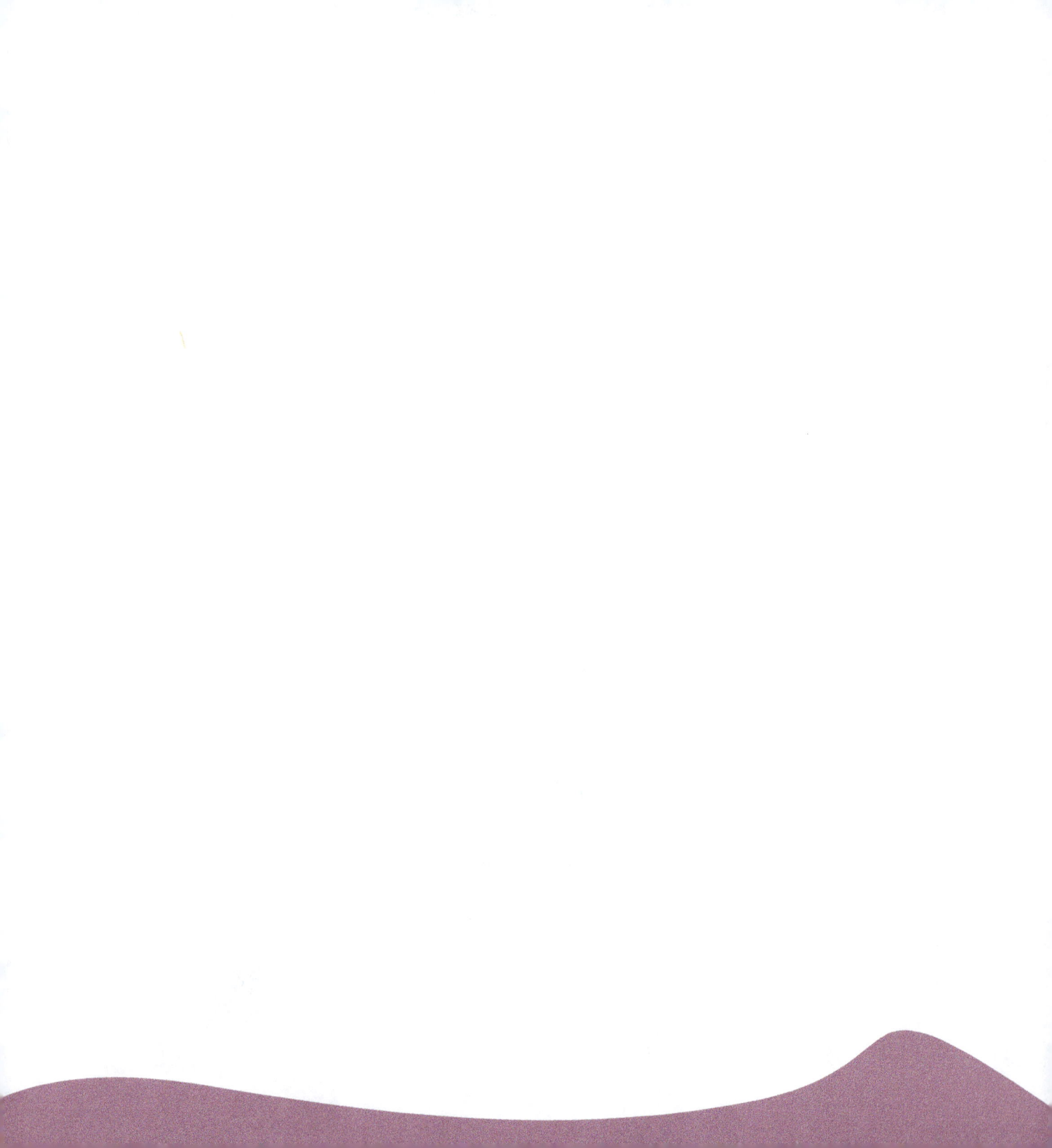

SAMANTHA VALE

FOREWORD BY DAME LAURA LEE CEO OF MAGGIES

The Lady WITH NO HAIR

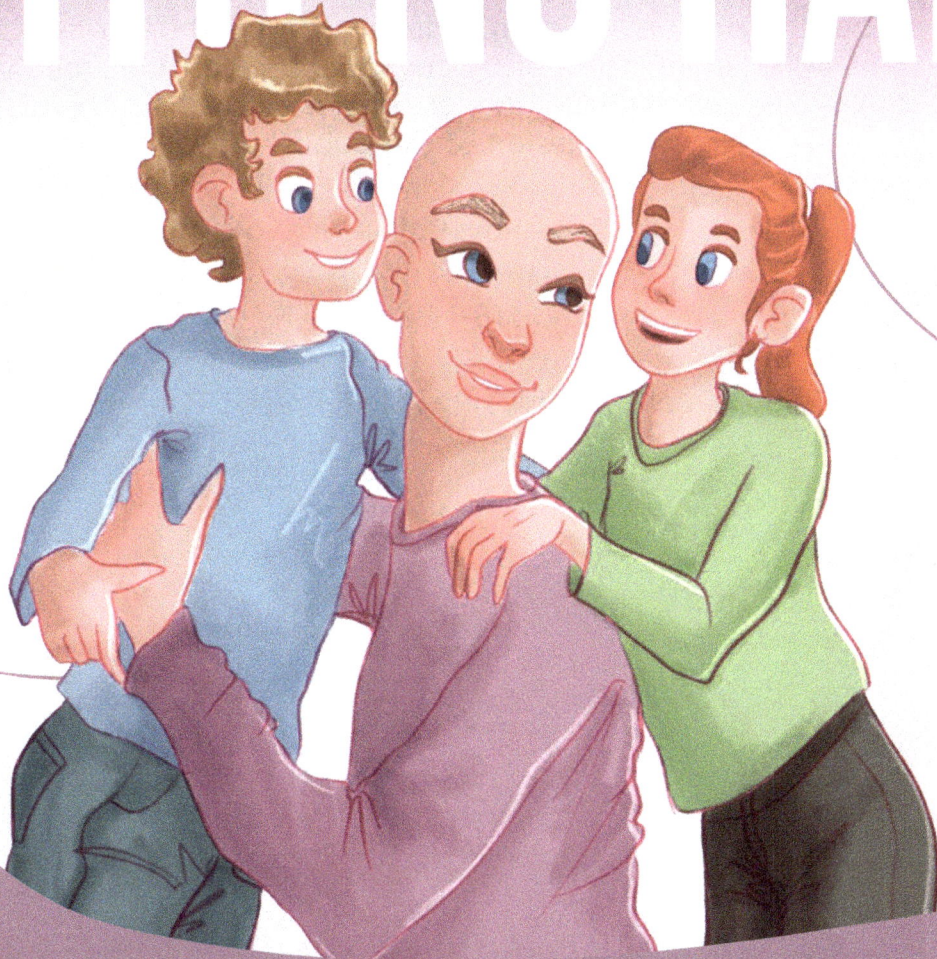

Illustrated by: Polina Nikolova

ISBN: 978-1-8382213-1-7

Published by: Tiny Angel Press LTD.

TINY ANGEL
Press Ltd

https://themonster-series.com

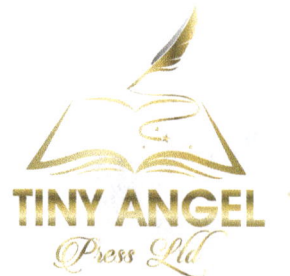

About the Author

My name is Sam and when I was 35 I was diagnosed with breast cancer. I underwent multiple surgeries, chemotherapy and radiotherapy over the course of 18 months and am now pleased to say that I am well and living life with a renewed sense of gratitude. Long may it last.

I am a mummy to Jack and Molly who were just six and four at the time of my diagnosis.

As with everything that life places in front of me, I try and find a way of making it make sense to my children.

Cancer doesn't make sense.

So I chose to try and use our experiences and turn them into something positive.

This is one of them.

We hope you enjoy our book.

Foreword

I love the honesty and affection in this beautifully written book about why hair loss in a parent can be so scary and difficult for a child.

Children grew up with stories, films and books about heroines with long thick hair and rarely see images of bald heads, especially in women, so it is very difficult when someone they love loses their hair. It can make them feel angry or afraid or embarrassed. At the same time they are trying to deal with someone they love being ill and life taking a different shape.

Talking about these issues can help so much and Samantha has done a brilliant job in raising them.

If you need support talking to your child about cancer we are always here to support you at Maggie's.

Maggies.org
Dame Laura Lee CEO of Maggies

My name is Jack.

I am 8 years old and live at home with my sister Molly, who is six and my mum.

Mum hasn't got any hair.

Let me tell you why.

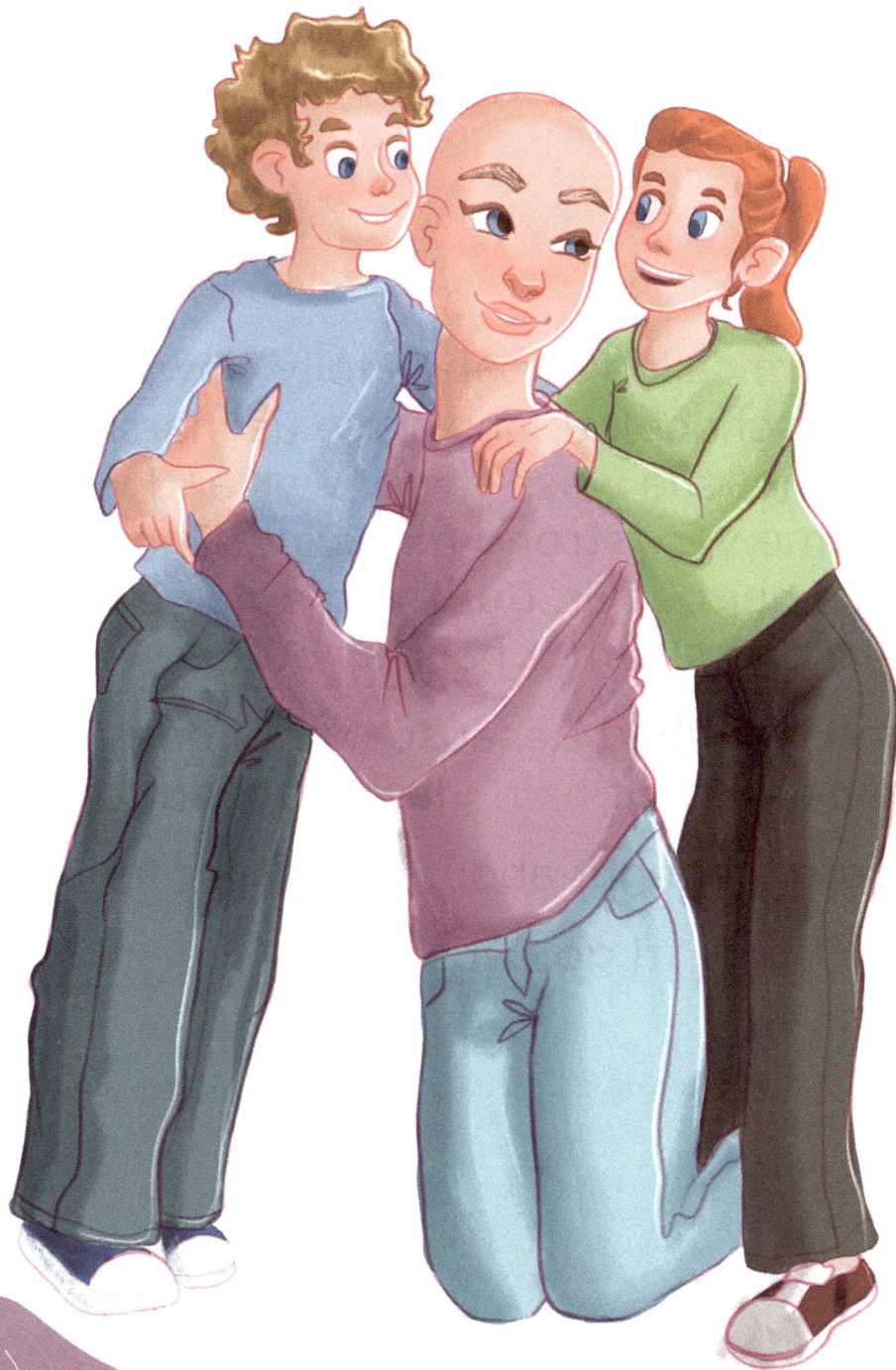

One day Mum called me and Molly downstairs. She made us hot chocolate and gave us marshmallows. She told us that she wasn't very well and would have to take some very strong medicine. The medicine would make her better. But the medicine would also make her hair fall out.

Molly and I laughed because it sounded funny. A mum without hair! Mum laughed too.

But the more I thought about it, the less funny it was.

I got worried.

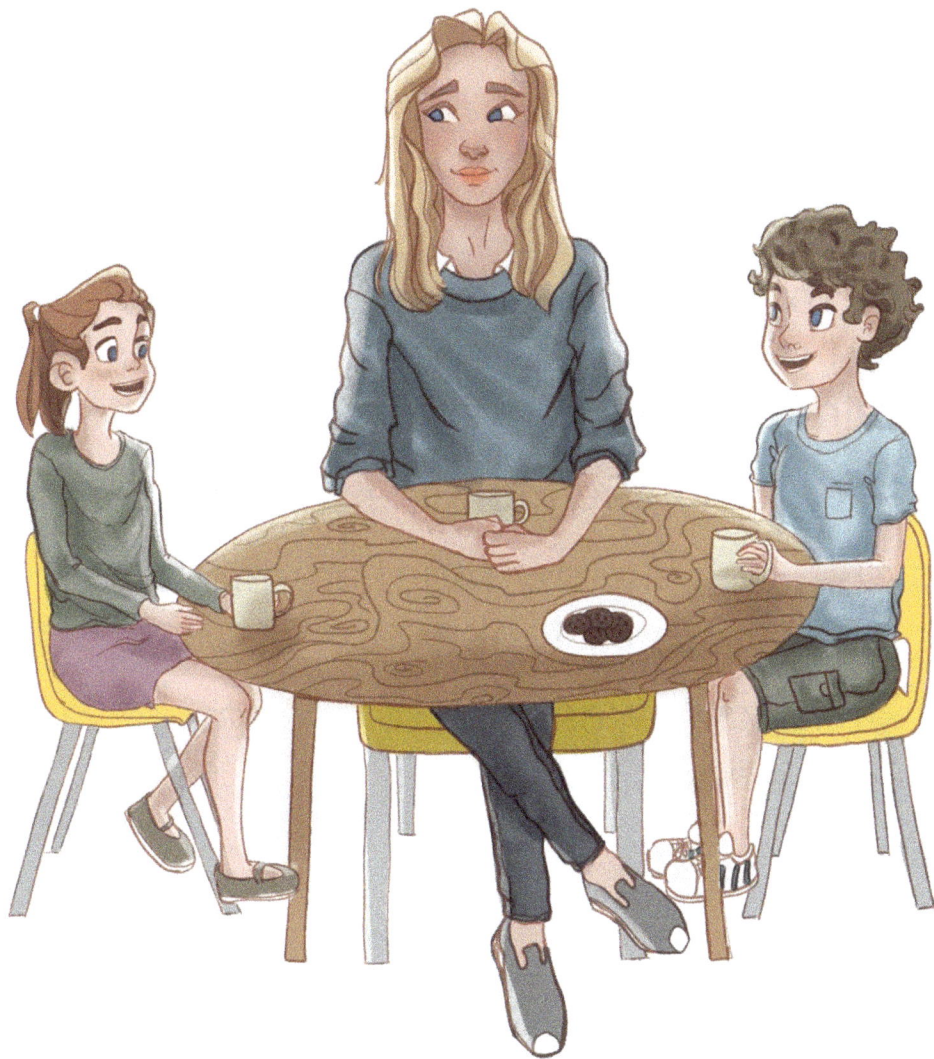

You see my mum had long flowing hair and it shimmered golden in the sunshine like a mermaid. When it rained it would go kind of fuzzy and wavy.

What would she look like with no hair?

She wouldn't look like my mum anymore. She might even look scary.

I didn't want her to change.

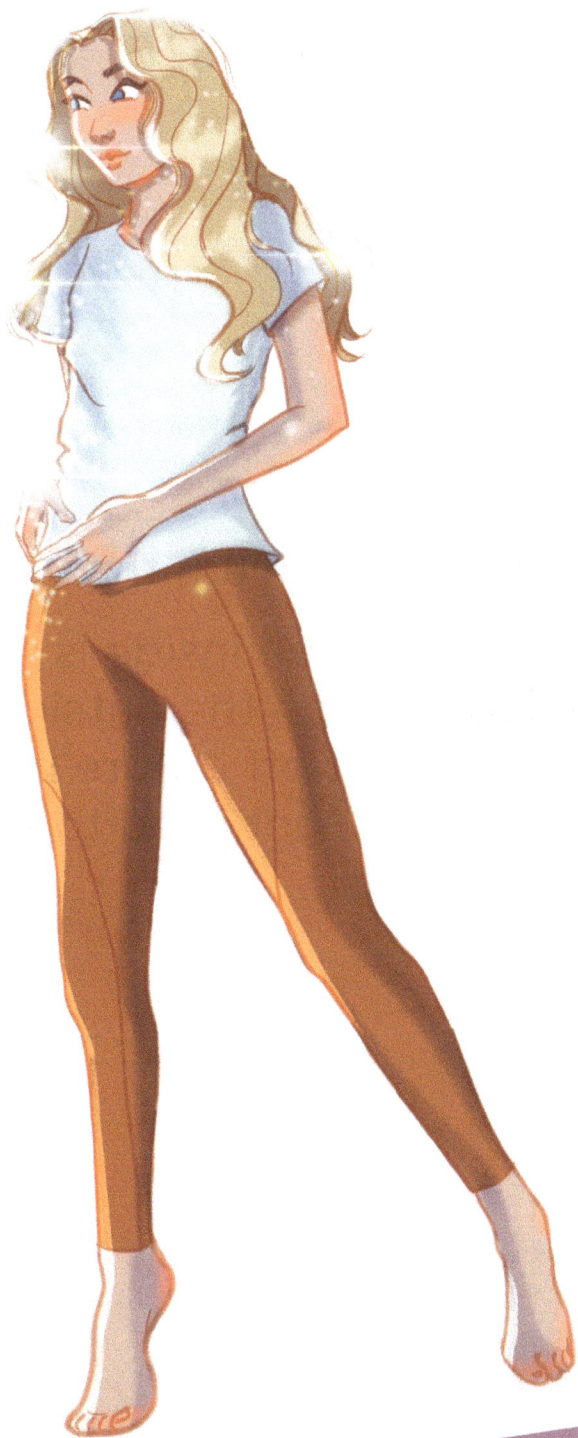

I tried to tell Mum that I was worried.

Mum said who we are inside is more important than what we look like on the outside. She said that she was going to cut it off before it fell out so we could get used to it.

I didn't want her to. But Mum kept saying, "Don't be silly Jack; it's only hair!"

I think she was a bit worried too. I sometimes heard her crying in the bathroom when she was brushing her hair.

'Maybe she just got some tangles," said Molly. "I get them sometimes."

A few days later, Mum came to wake me up to get ready for school. She had a hat on her head. "I cut my hair very short," she said. "Would you like to see?"

I shut my eyes tight. Mum said that it was OK if I didn't want to see it but that sooner or later I would have to.

I rolled over and buried my face in my pillow.

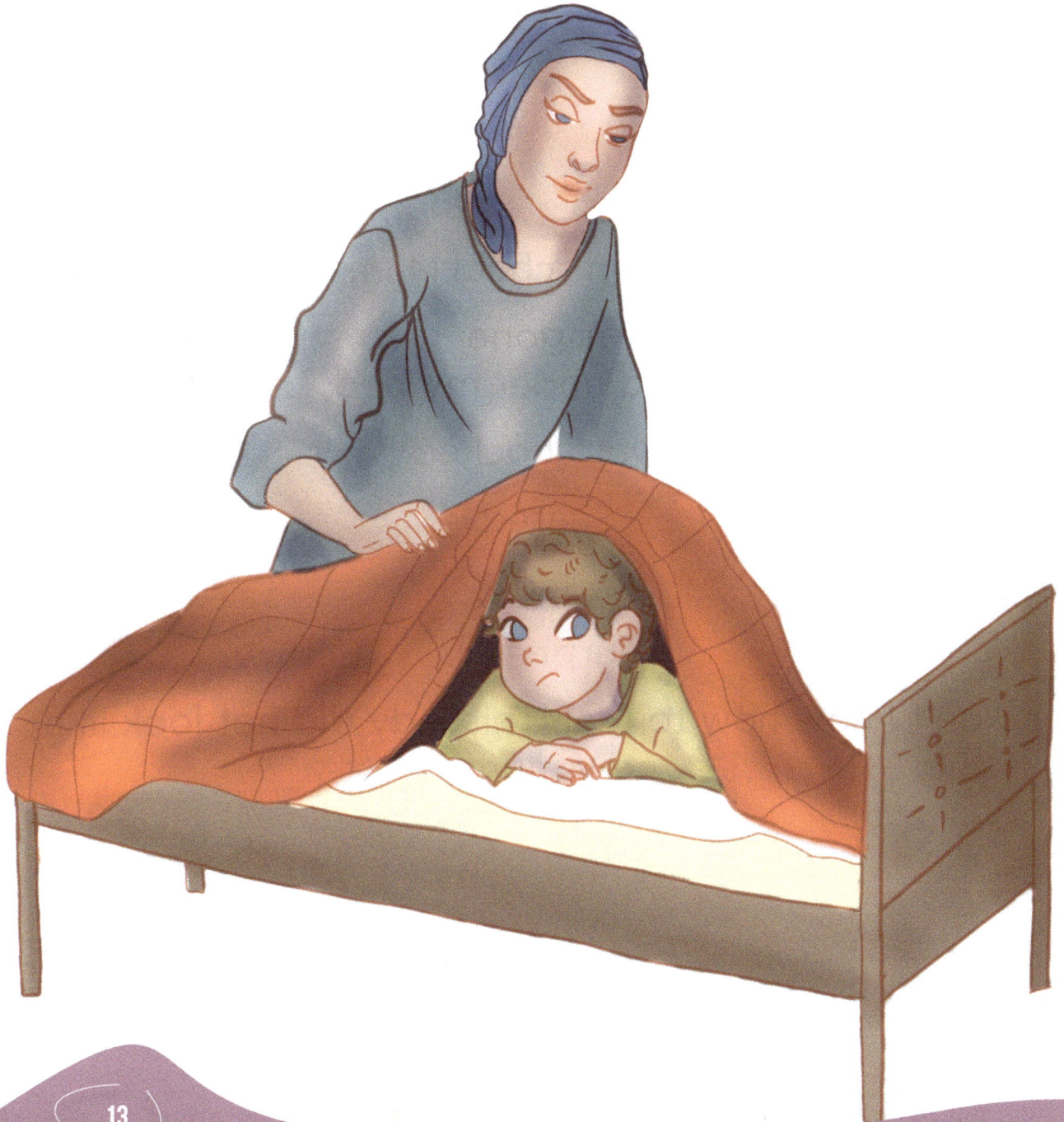

When I came home from school Mum took her hat off.

Mum's mermaid hair was gone! I ran straight upstairs and hid under my bed.

I was shocked.

Scared.

Sad.

Surprised.

I didn't know how to feel. This lady did not look like my mum.

Mum said, "Hold my hands Jack. Look into my eyes. Don't look at my head, just my eyes".

So I did.

I looked at her eyes until I saw my mum again.

She said that over the next few weeks the short hair would fall out. When that started to happen, she would shave it all off. Then she would be completely bald.

The first time that Mum took us to school, she asked us if we wanted her to wear something to cover her head. Molly said, "No!" She was excited and wanted her friends to see Mum with no hair.

I didn't want my friends to see my hairless mum that didn't look like my mum anymore. So Mum put a hat on in the car.

I don't think many people noticed that Mum was bald to begin with because she wore hats and scarves.

I hated Mum taking me to school but I hated her picking me up afterwards even more. Dropping off was quick, I didn't want her to kiss me goodbye in front of my friends so would kiss her in the car and then jump out really quickly and dash in.

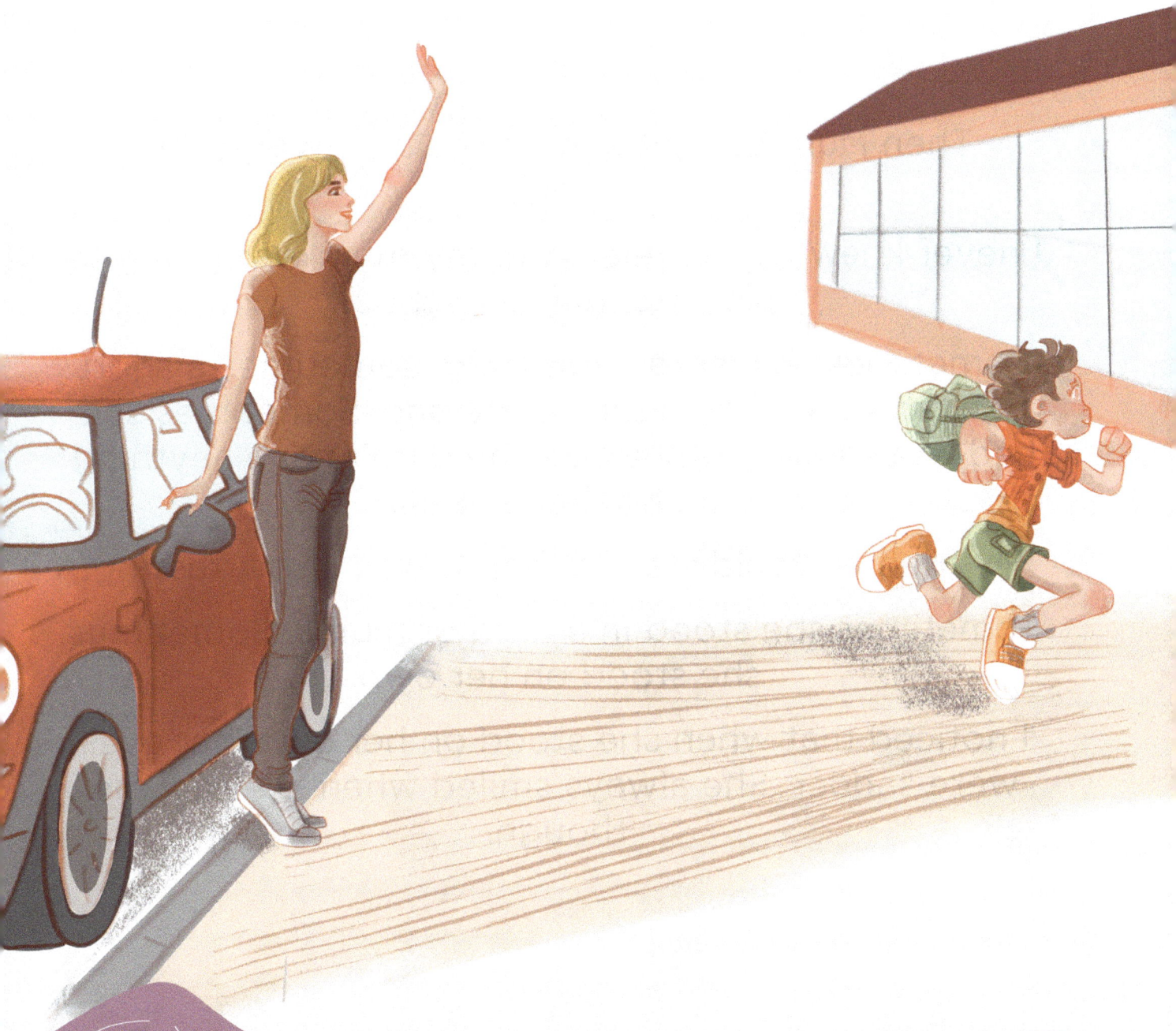

Then Mum bought some wigs and everything changed.

I never knew which version of my mum was going to pick me up from school.

Sometimes she wore a long wig, sometimes a short one. She even had a pink curly one. Sometimes she had a scarf and sometimes she didn't have anything on her head at all.

My friends would stare at her. It was embarrassing.

Sometimes she stood in a herd of mums. Sometimes she stood on her own.

I noticed that when she stood on her own, her eyes were sadder. She always smiled when she saw me though.

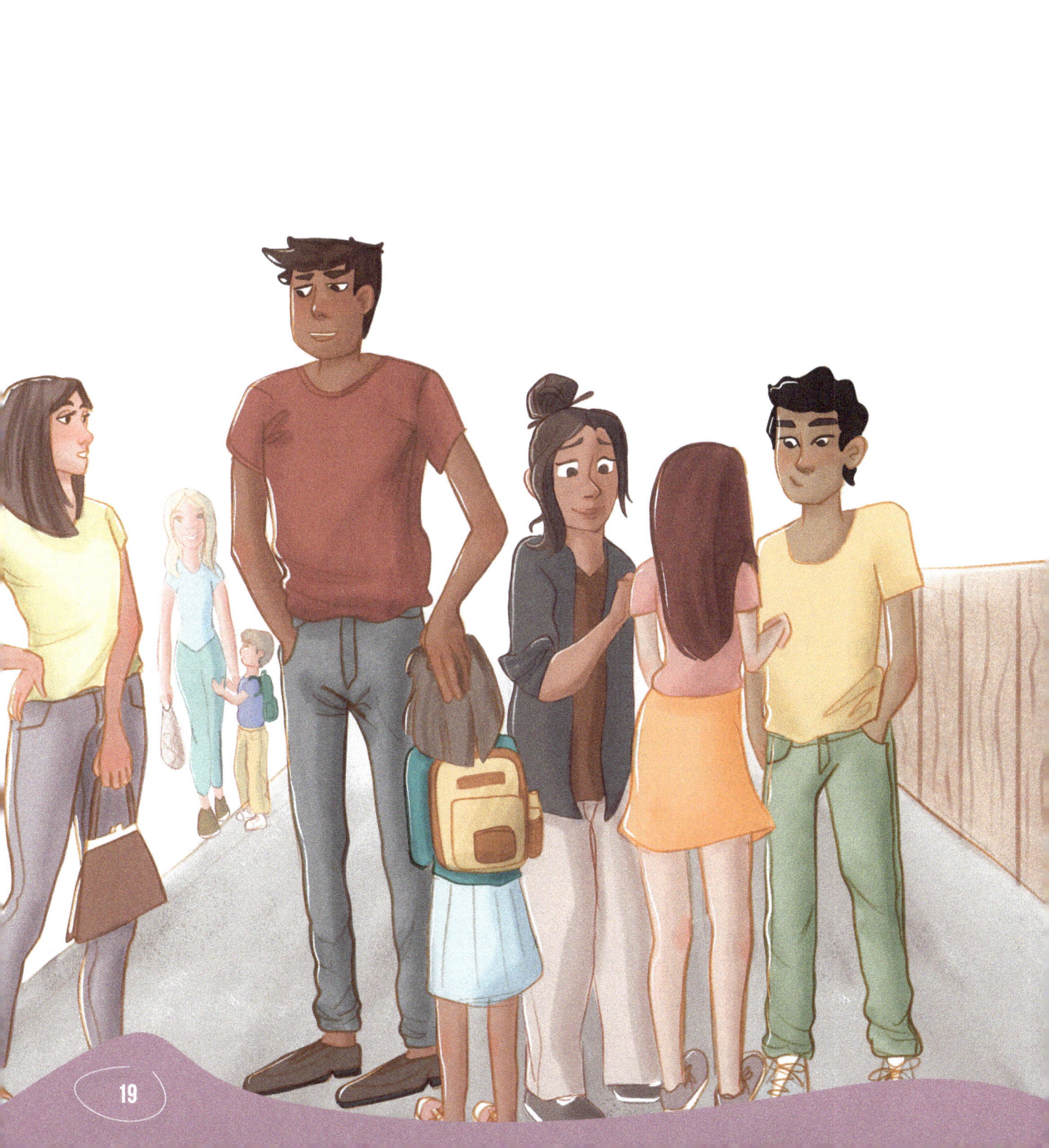

As the weeks passed, Mum wore wigs and hats more and more. She didn't mind people staring at her. But winter can be chilly and it's nice to have a warm head. Grandpa says the same thing, he always wears hats when it's cold outside and he is bald too. So it must be true.

I remember one day we went to the sweet shop in town and Mum went out without a hat, scarf or a wig. I got strawberry laces and Molly had chocolate buttons. In the queue, I overheard a girl behind us.

"Mum, is that a man or a lady?"

I don't know what the girl's mum said but I felt myself getting hotter. Of course it was a lady! It was my mum.

"Where is her hair? Ladies have hair."

I felt tears sting my eyes. I wanted to turn around and give this girl a shove. I was angry at my mum. Why couldn't she just be normal like the other mums? Look normal. Act normal. I really missed her long, mermaid hair.

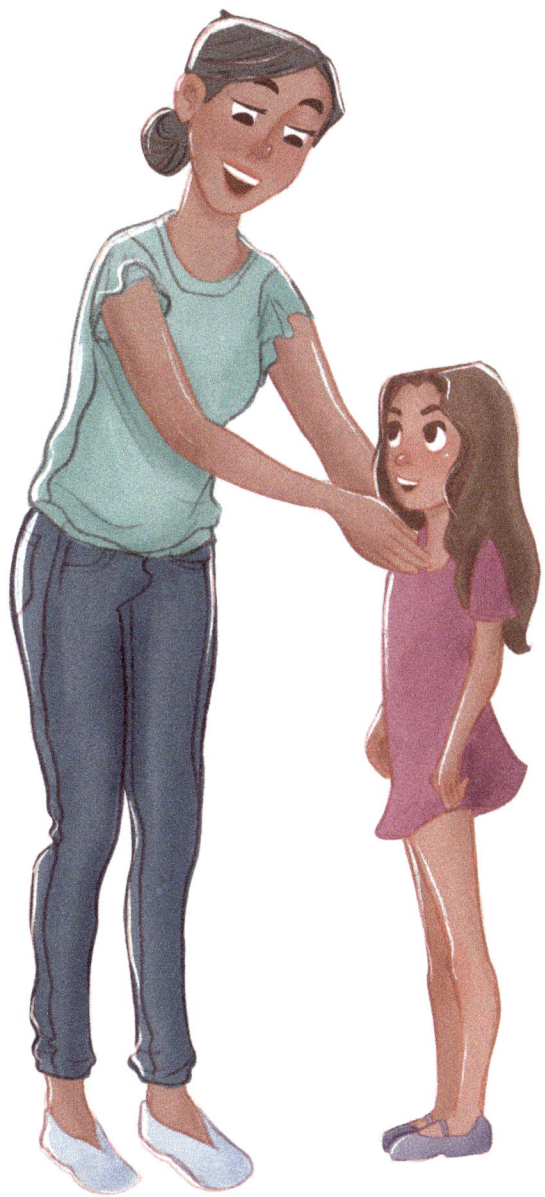

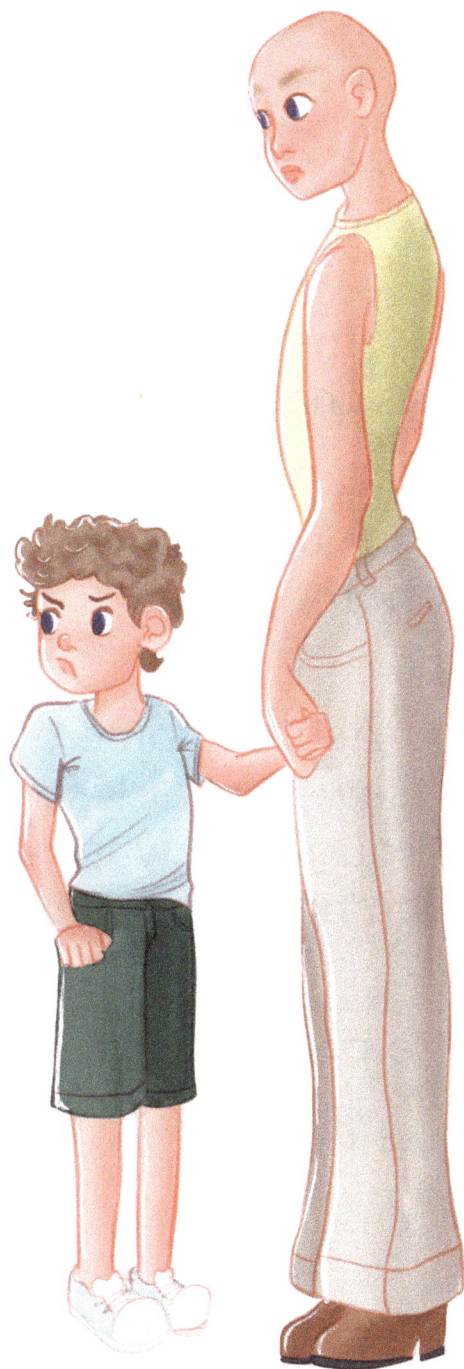

Mum normally stays bald when we are at home. She says that wigs make her head hot and itchy if she wears them for too long.

I got used to seeing Mum with no hair. When we were at home it was normal. I sometimes forgot that it wasn't normal for other people.

Ashton came over to play the other day. Ashton saw my hairless mum but he didn't say anything. I thought he was going to ask me why and I would feel embarrassed – but he didn't, and I didn't. Maybe his mum had told him already?

We played with Lego and had fish fingers for tea. It felt normal.

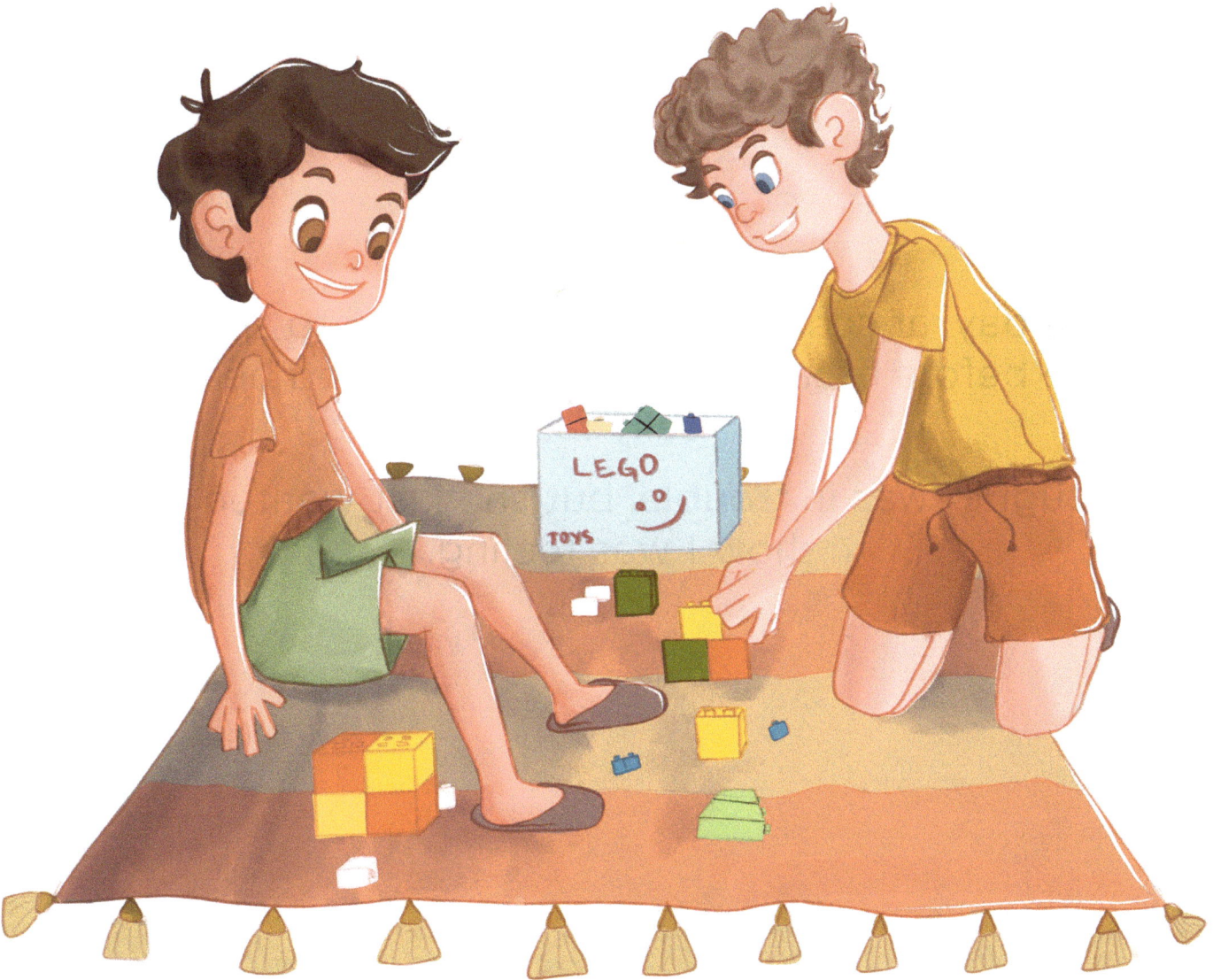

One day, at school, the teacher asked to speak to me before break time. My heart started beating really fast.

I thought I was in trouble, but she just wanted to ask how I was feeling.

I don't really know what to say when a grown-up asks me how I am feeling. Sometimes I feel happy, sometimes sad. Sometimes angry and sometimes like there is a pit in my stomach, so deep that I can't feel the bottom. Sometimes I don't even know what I feel.

So I just say, "I'm fine." Most grown-ups seem OK with that response.

We went into London to celebrate Chinese New Year and Mum wore one of her wigs. It was really busy. Molly was on Mum's shoulders and I was holding Mum's hand. There were so many people! We were all crammed together in really narrow streets, with dragons, drums, decorations and noise everywhere. As Molly climbed down from Mum's shoulders, she lost her balance and pulled off Mum's wig by mistake! Luckily Mum thought it was funny. She just put the wig in her backpack and we carried on watching the dancing dragons.

I actually saw a few bald ladies that day.

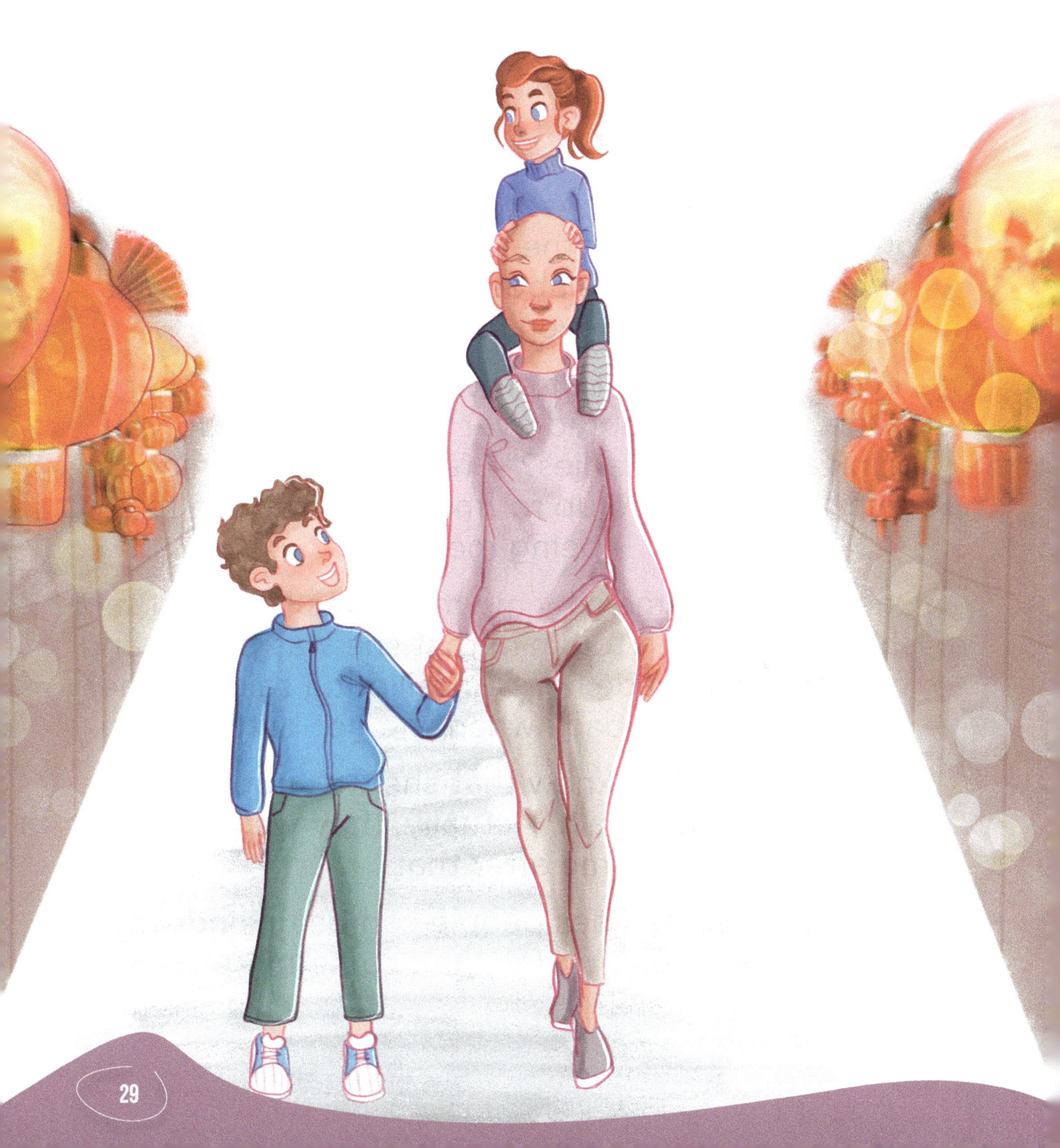

One day at school, Ashton and I were playing at break time. Some of the kids in the year above me were making a joke about bald people. It wasn't even funny.

I could hear them but pretended to ignore them. One of them shouted over to me, "What do you think about bald ladies?" I felt my face burning up again. Ashton stood up for me and told them to stop being mean.

One boy asked me why my mum was bald and said she looked silly. I told him that she was poorly and her medicine made her hair fall out. I said that her hair would grow back when she got better again.

I don't think they knew that she was poorly. They didn't tease me again. Actually, they were nicer to me after that.

Mum says sometimes people can be unkind when they don't understand something.

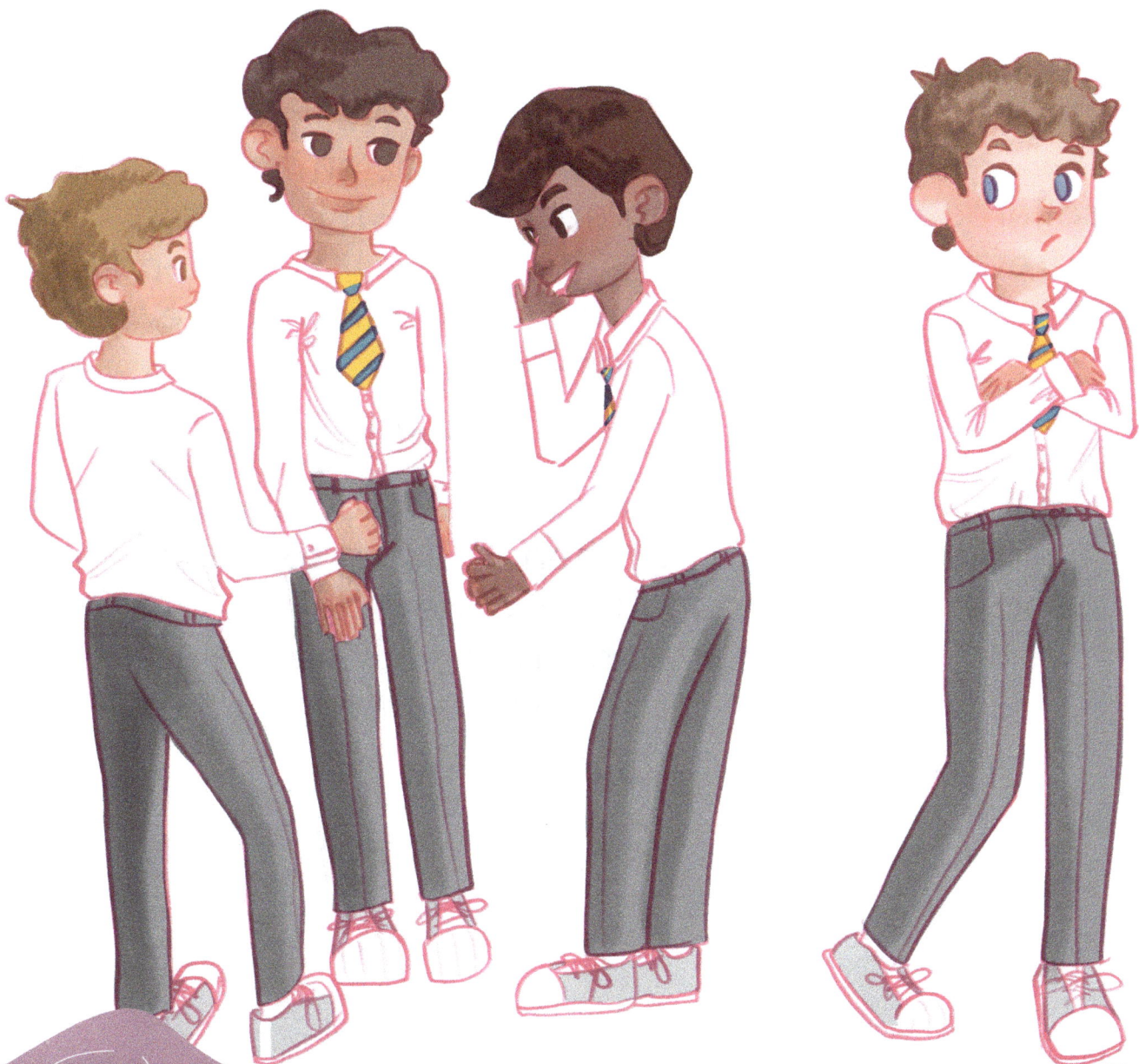

There was this really funny time when we were at a theme park and Mum was feeling well enough after taking so much medicine. We went on a really scary rollercoaster that hung upside down in the air! I am pretty sure that Mum didn't know it was going to do that because I am sure she wouldn't have worn her wig.

It flew off in the middle of the ride!

Mum screamed and then started laughing. I didn't know what to do but then I started to laugh too and everyone around us got the giggles! But they weren't laughing at Mum. They were laughing *with* Mum because she was laughing too!

I can't explain how I knew this. I just knew.

That was a great day.

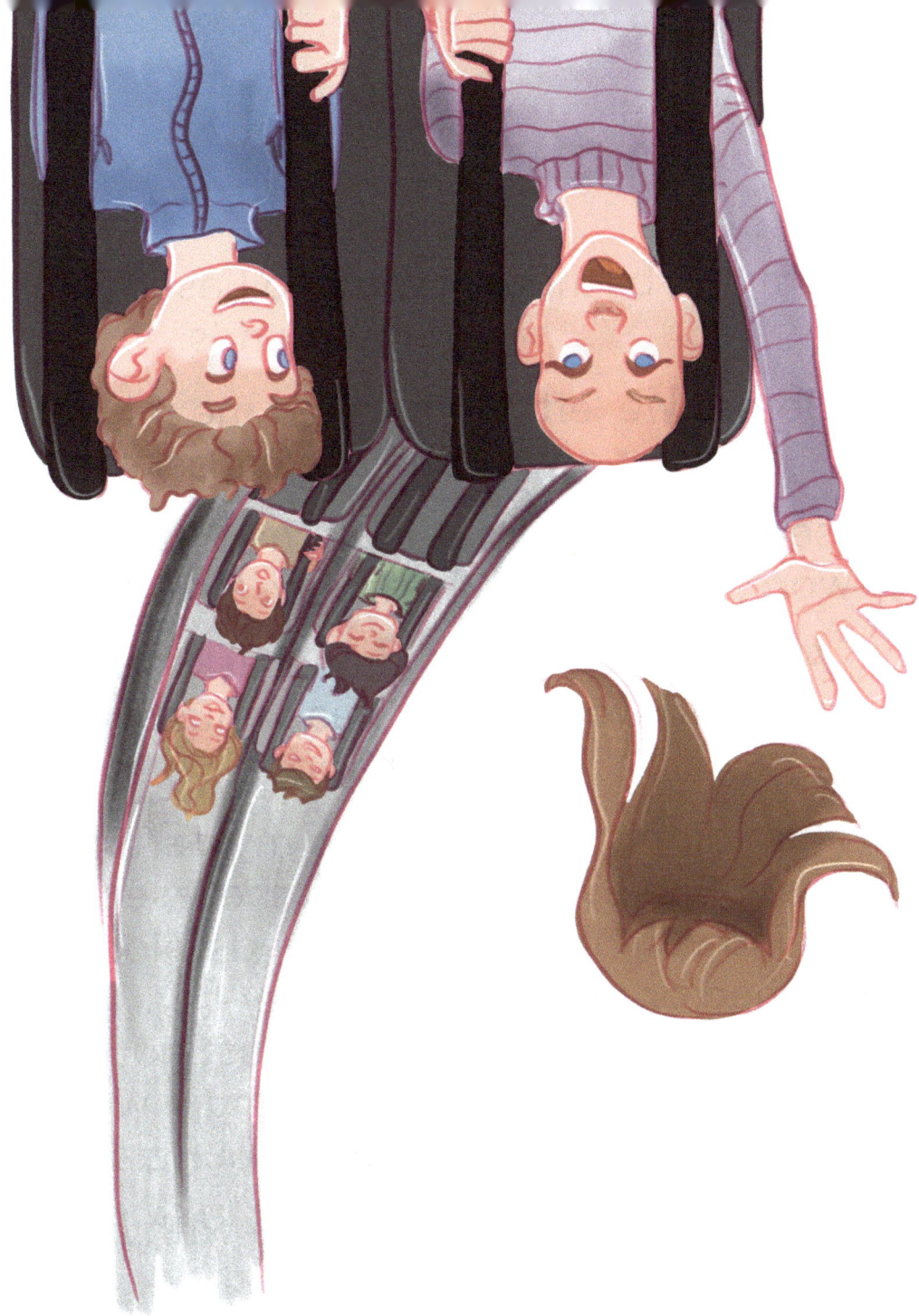

For my 8th birthday, I went to Laser Quest with some of my friends.

Before we left, Mum asked me if I wanted her to wear a wig. She always asks me that.

I used to worry about it all the time. But I don't really worry anymore. When I say, "I feel fine," I mean it.

And so, for the first time, I asked Mum what *she* wanted to wear on her head. I just wanted her to be happy.

Mum didn't wear a wig to my party. Or a hat, or a scarf. She even came into the laser arena and ran around with me and my friends. None of my friends laughed or made fun of me or her. They never even said anything. They were just normal and cool. Kameron even said that my mum was probably the coolest mum in our class.

I definitely agree with him.

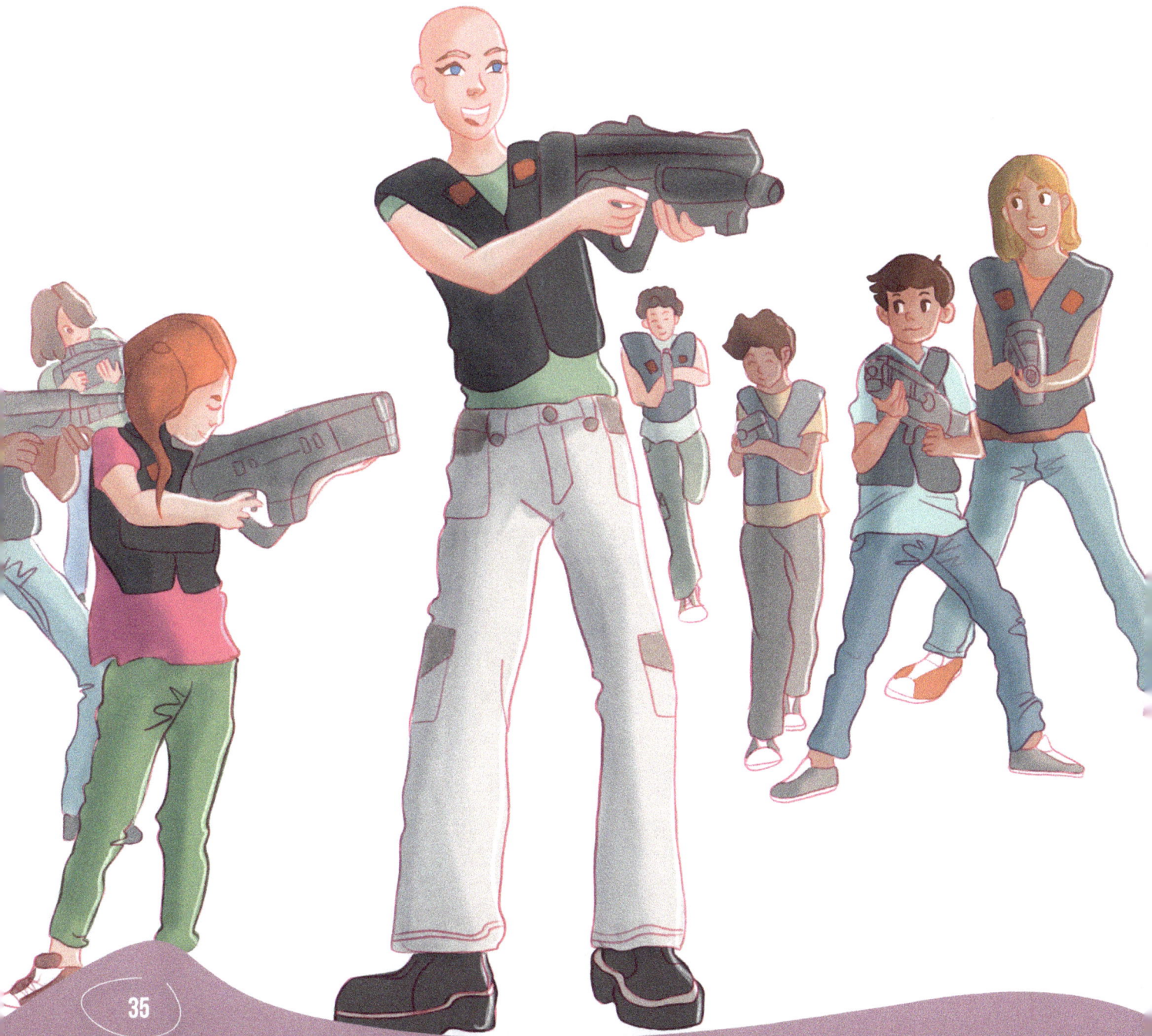

My name is Jack and my mum hasn't got any hair.

She said it will grow back. I don't really mind anymore.

I love her anyway.

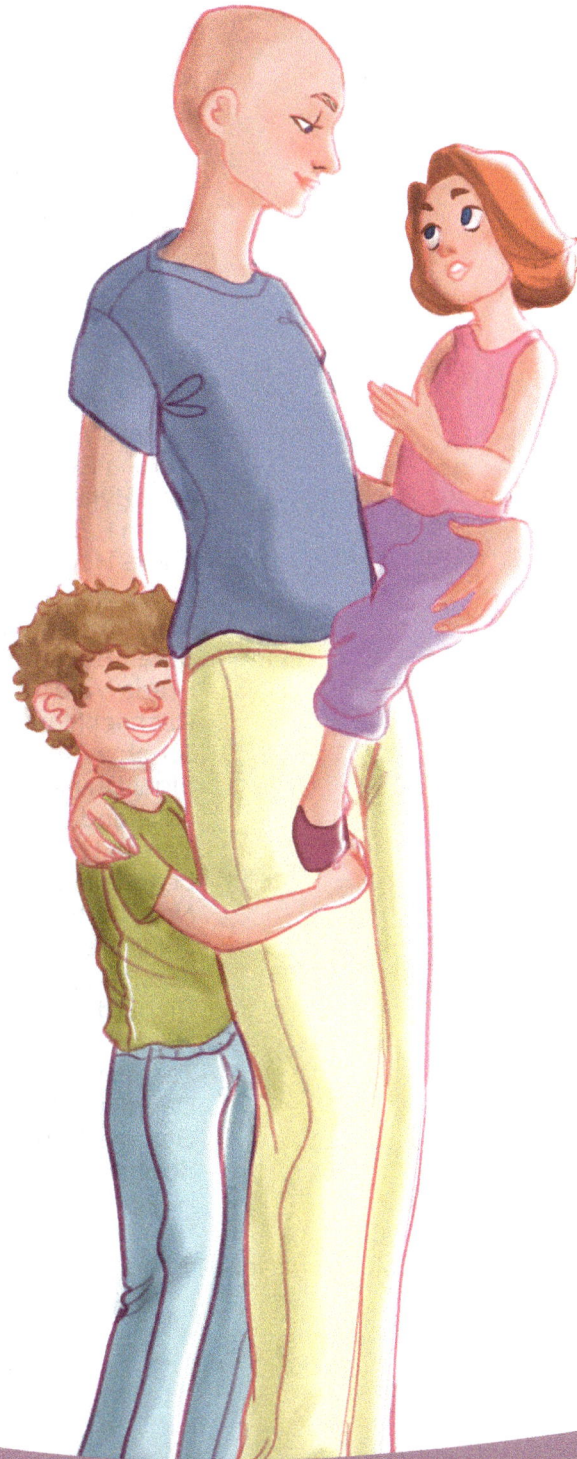

THANKS TO THE PEOPLE THAT MADE THIS BOOK POSSIBLE:

Elena Gilbert
Lee Bright
Stef King
Andrew Fowler
Gabriella Reisinger
Amy Butterfield
Amy Deane
Philip Allinson
Kirstie Scott
Christine Findlay
Valerie Hewison
Natalie Woods
Carol Miles
Lesley Anne Bremner
Bobbie Chatt
Sarah Bacon
Andy Green
Elizabeth Purcell
Matt Lunn
Rosalind Cox
Stephen and Lesley Vale
Karen Bartlett
Amanda Green
Miss Yvonne Plester
Marina Trigg
Claire Van den Berg
Kate Rodman
Natasha Nugent
Chris Wood
Jackie Beaven
Hayley Chapman
Lucy Harman
Vicky and Giles Stoakley
Caroline Morgan
Lizzie Constantine
Marie Mcdermott

Karen Hobbs
Emma and Chris
Susan Dumbarton
Lisa Allen and The Pink Foundation
David Hynes
Rachel McCourty
Jackie Crewe
Nicky Short
Claire Smith
Caroline Sturman
Sam Ormerod Shaw
Sophie Wheater
Amelia Reimink
Ann Hyland
Helen R Shead
Laura Harriet Bailey
Abby Malton
Saffron Honour
Sarah Bevan
Freda Vale
Rachael Maxwell
Stephanie Raper
Sigal Duvshani-Eli
Julie and Adi Vale
Teresa Hall
Leanne McGrath
Naz Akhter
Julie Green
Jessica Spanier
Richard Curtis
Helen W. Jarrett
Tanya Mason
David and Val Thomson
Gemma Cholerton
Sophie Pearce
Helen Frewin

Also a huge thank you to Steve Cole for his input in editing.

www.ingramcontent.com/pod-product-compliance
Lightning Source LLC
Chambersburg PA
CBHW080148310326
41914CB00090B/904